Diabetes
- Guide -

Prevention and Management For This Global Lifestyle Disease

RON KNESS

Contents

Disclaimer

We hope you enjoy reading our report, however we do suggest you read our disclaimer. All the material written in this document is provided for informational purposes only and is general in nature.

Every person is a unique individual and what has worked for some or even many may not work for you. Any information perceived as advice by must be considered in light of your own particular set of circumstances.

 The author or person sharing this information does not assume any responsibility for the accuracy or outcome of your use of the content.

 Every attempt has been made to provide well researched and up to date content at the time of writing.

Now all the legalities have been taken care of, please enjoy the content.

See your healthcare professional before starting any diet, health or exercise program!

Introduction

One of the best ways to stay healthy is to stay informed. Certainly, knowing more about insulin and blood glucose is a must not only for all diabetics but for their family members too. Typically, if one family member has diabetes it will impact the rest of the family and they will have to make some adjustments – especially in their eating habits.

Significantly, statistics indicate that if Type 2 diabetes hasn't affected you or your family already, it will, sooner or later. Diabetes is becoming a global epidemic. Type 2 diabetes is on the rise even among small children.

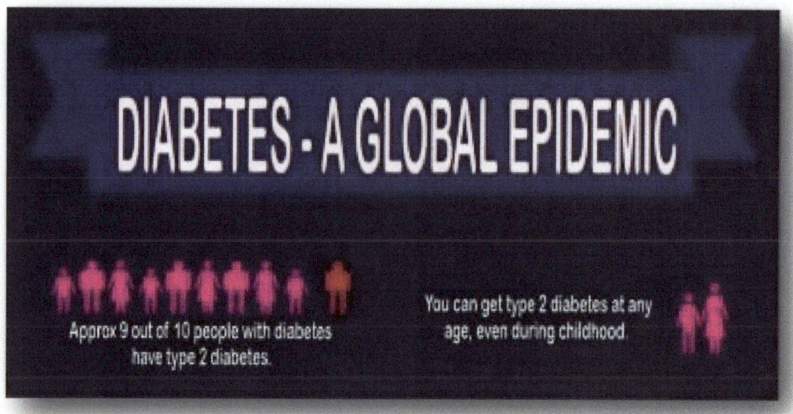

Modern lifestyles – predominantly food choices, but also eating and exercising behaviors – means a conscious and mindful effort is required to avoid the seemingly inevitable progression from overweight, through obesity and pre-diabetes to full-blown Type 2, with all its health risks.

It is most important to realize that being diagnosed with Type 2 diabetes is not the end of your world. We do have control, if we choose to exercise it. And because Type 2 diabetes is a result of a poor lifestyle, it can be controlled and even reversed once positive lifestyle changes are made. Look at your diet and your lifestyle and that of your family. Make the changes now before it is too late.

It is important to understand how our food choices affect insulin release and how it impacts our overall health.

Prevention and management starts at home … with you. Understanding a few factors in this guide is a good beginning.

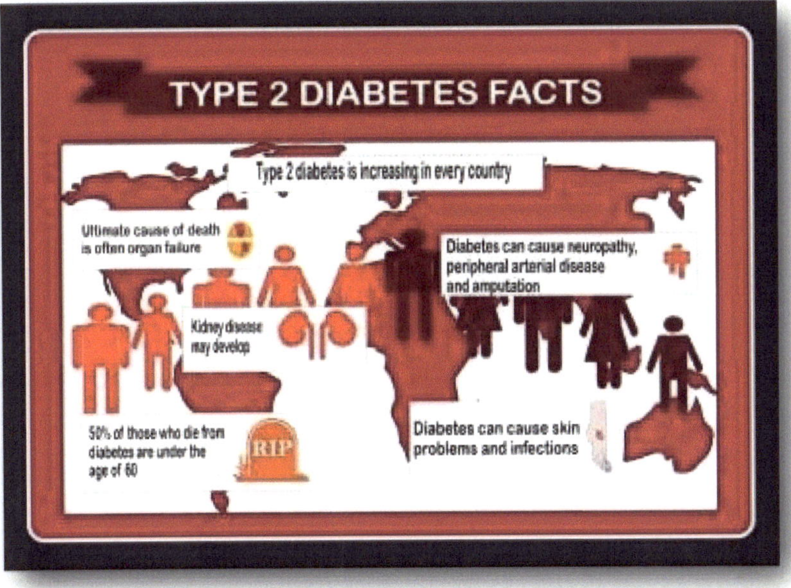

Hyperglycemia vs. Hypoglycemia

Hyperglycemia also spelled Hyperglycaemia, refers to having abnormally high blood sugar. The prefix "hyper" translates to "high." The main symptoms of this condition include extreme thirst or polydipsia and frequent urination or polyuria.

Hyperglycaemia is a symptom that occurs in both Type 1 and Type 2 Diabetes.

In a healthy functioning body, the pancreas normally releases insulin after a meal to enable the cells of the body to utilize glucose for energy. In a non-diabetic, this fluctuation keeps glucose levels in a healthy range.

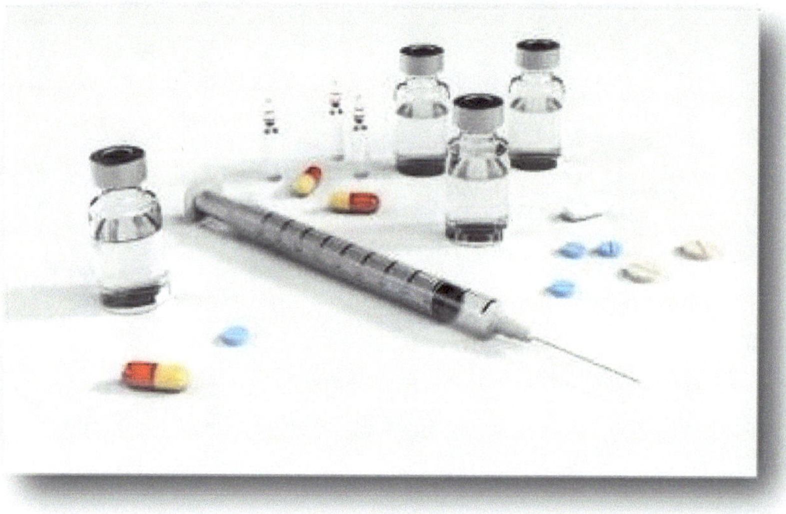

However with diabetes, the blood sugar levels become severely elevated. This can result in a medical emergency such as HHNS or hyperglycemia hyperosmolar state. Diabetic ketoacidosis or DKA can also be another severe consequence that can result from the body trying to cope with too much glucose.

Symptoms and Signs of Hyperglycemia

Diabetes is the main cause of hyperglycemia; however, there are other medical conditions that may cause this condition to present including: Pancreatitis, Hyperthyroidism, Pancreatic cancer, Cushing's syndrome, unusual tumors that secrete hormones, severe illnesses and certain medications.

The long-term effects of hyperglycemia can be quite dramatic. Often, these issues develop slowly over a period of years, especially in diabetics who are not effectively managing their health properly.

Some key complications include: heart and blood vessel disease, which can increase the risk of peripheral artery disease, stroke, and heart attack. Nerve damage is another potential problem that can lead to tingling, pain and burning sensations. Gum disease and eye diseases including damage to the retina, cataracts and glaucoma are also prevalent.

Hypoglycemia

Hypoglycemia or hypoglycaemia on the other hand, is a medical emergency of diminished blood glucose or excessively low blood sugar. The prefix "hypo" translates to "low." Also referred to as "Hyperinsulinism," low blood sugar levels result from overstimulation of insulin in the pancreas.

The pancreas eventually becomes exhausted from releasing insulin too frequently in order to combat the high levels of sugar present in the blood.

Symptoms and Signs of Hypoglycemia

Symptoms of hypoglycemia can vary greatly, however, the main concern are issues arising from an inadequate supply of glucose to the brain. Hypoglycemic manifestations can be divided into the following: Adrenergic manifestations due to falling glucose; lack of glucose in the brain resulting in neuroglycopenic symptoms; and glucagon manifestations.

Neuroglycopenic effects due to a shortage of glucose in the brain can cause a severe impairment of function, known as neuroglycopenia. Neuroglycopenic symptoms can range from dizziness, tiredness, weakness, blurred vision, confusion and difficulty concentrating. Inappropriate behavior can also occur that may be mistaken for intoxication. In severe cases, seizures, unconsciousness, coma and even death can occur.

Many people consider themselves to be "hypoglycemic." Typically, these individuals are referring to symptoms triggered by falling glucose adrenergic manifestations. This condition may present with anxiety, shakiness, coldness, dilated pupils, nervousness, tachycardia or rapid heartbeat and palpitations. Paresthesia or feeling of "pins and needles" or numbness is also commonly experienced. Immediately consuming some orange juice or candy can usually remedy this uncomfortable situation.

Glucagon manifestations of hypoglycemia may present with the following: abdominal discomfort; vomiting; hunger, stomach rumbling or borborygmus and headache.

There are some great ways you can be proactive with your diet and eating habits. Becoming educated on the glycemic index and starting to read food labels are great places to start. Try some new recipes and think positive about re-learning your relationship with food.

Glycemic Index - Diet and Diabetes

The Glycemic Index or Glycaemic Index, often referred to as GI, can a useful tool for diabetics. It can be helpful for practically anyone who wishes to educate themselves on how quickly glucose levels in the blood rise after eating a certain kind of food.

This index provides numerical values for foods. You can easily use the Internet at home or on your phone to find out the glycemic index of a particular food. The GI estimates how much each gram of available carbohydrate, which is the total carbohydrate without the fiber content, in a food raises a person's blood sugar level after they eat it. This measurement is relative to consumption of pure glucose, which has its own glycemic index of 100. The higher the number the more impact that food will have on your blood sugar level.

One of the things to take into consideration with the glycemic index is that it does not factor in the actual amount of carbohydrate that is consumed in the serving. The Glycemic Load however, a related measure, takes this into account by multiplying the carbohydrate content of the actual serving by the glycemic index of the particular food.

Foods that are considered to be Low GI measure in at 55 or less. Medium GI foods are considered to be 56-69 and High Glycemic Index foods measure at 70 and above.

Understanding your portion size or the amount of food you are eating per serving and how fast this food will be broken down into glucose, will enable you to make wiser food choices.

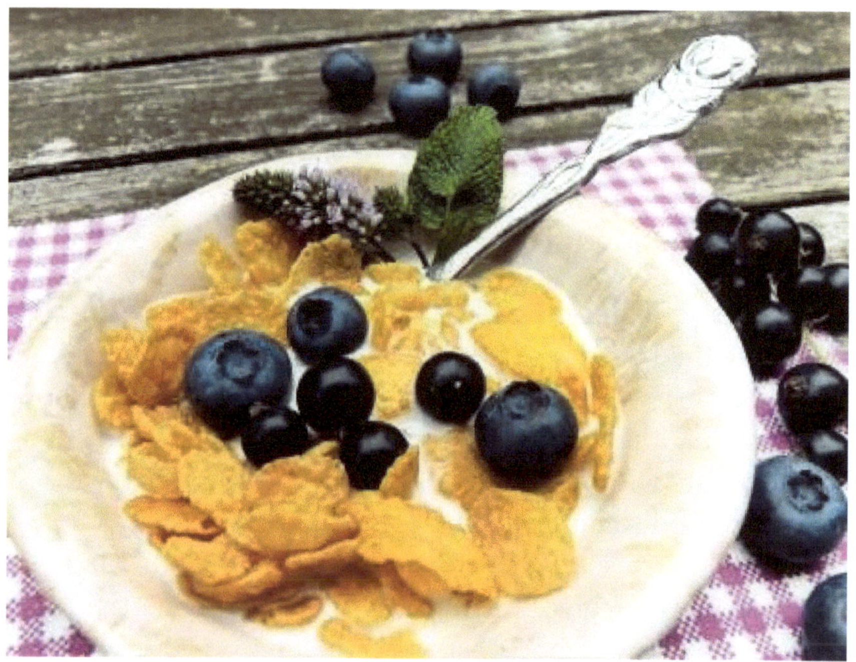

If you do want that extra glass of wine or piece of chocolate cake, you will be able to calculate the rest of your daily meals to ensure you are balancing your carbohydrate intake safely.

Avoid High Glycemic Foods

We all know, or need to know, that sweets and processed foods are not healthy. Carbohydrates which break down easily during digestion and rapidly release glucose into our bloodstream are high glycemic foods.

Be wary of pure fruit juices, salad dressings, condiments, health bars and cereals, white rice, potatoes, white bread, ice cream, chocolate, oranges and bananas. These foods are all considered to be on the higher side of the glycemic index.

Be sure to read labels on condiments, sauces and pre-packaged foods. Even many foods we grew up considering to be healthy can lead you astray. Proportion is everything.

Also note that ingredients are listed in the order of abundance; the first ingredient being the most prominent all the way down to the least.

Oftentimes the "pure or natural" ingredient advertised on the packaging will be way down on the bottom of the list! Be a smart consumer. If you have never previously read your food labels, now is the time to start. Your blood sugar and the rest of your body will thank you for taking the time!

Examples of Low Glycemic Foods

Carbohydrates that break down slower and release sugar more gradually into the bloodstream are considered to be low glycemic foods. Wholegrain bread, oats, barley, millet, wheat germ, lentils, baked halibut, soybeans and most beans are some popular choices.

Peaches, strawberries, mangoes, pumpkin seeds, sunflower seeds, peanuts, and most vegetables are also great choices.

What is Diabetes Mellitus?

Diabetes is a condition that results in high blood sugar (glucose) levels in the body. When the pancreas does not secrete enough insulin, high blood sugar levels result.

This may occur for one of two reasons: either the pancreas is not making enough insulin or the cells are unresponsive to the insulin that is being produced. Excess glucose in the blood is eliminated in the urine via the kidneys.

Insulin, a peptide hormone, is produced by the beta cells in our pancreas and is responsible for helping certain cells in the body absorb glucose or blood sugar and convert it into energy. Therefore, insulin is crucial in regulating fat and carbohydrate metabolism within our body.

Once control of insulin levels fail, the blood glucose or blood sugar level in the body can reach dangerously high levels, and Diabetes mellitus can result. This disease is a chronic disorder of carbohydrate, protein and fat metabolism.

If left untreated, this condition can have detrimental effects to your level of well-being. Many vital organs, including the heart and your circulatory system, the kidneys and the eyes and even your arms and legs may be adversely affected.

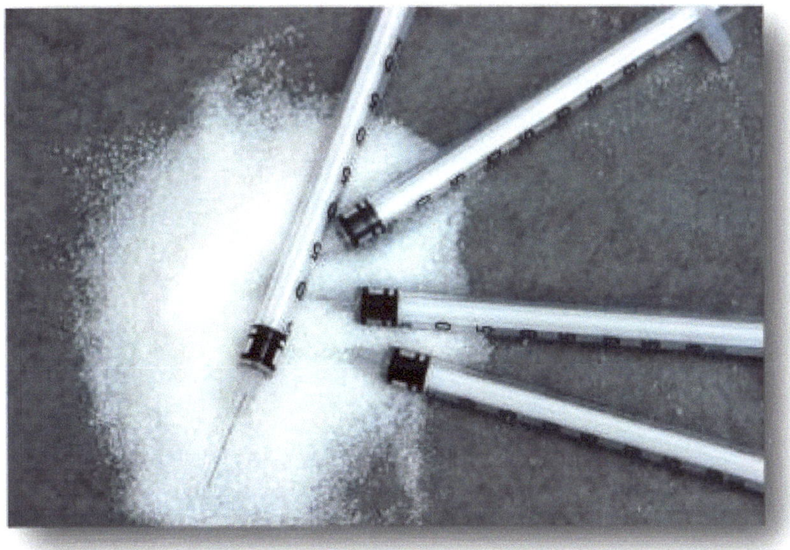

Symptoms of Diabetes

There are 3 classical symptoms of Diabetes, which may be remembered as the 3P's:

- Polydipsia or frequent thirst
- Polyuria or frequent urination
- Polyphagia or frequent hunger

Additional symptoms to be aware of include:

- Severe weight loss or emaciation can occur despite being excessively hungry
- Skin ulcers that appear anywhere on the body and are slow to heal
- Weakness
- Boils
- Loss of tactile sensation in the fingertips

- In women, there may be itching of the vulvae present
- In men there may be inflammation of the glans penis

Having continually elevated levels of blood glucose can cause changes in the shape of the lens in the eye, due to glucose absorption in the lens itself. This can result in vision changes and many people complain of blurred vision prior to being diagnosed with diabetes.

Diabetic dermadromes is a term describing a collective number of cutaneous conditions of the skin that are also commonly experienced by patients who have had diabetes for some time.

Different Types of Diabetes

There are three main kinds of diabetes mellitus: Type 1 DM, Type 2 DM and Gestational Diabetes. Other kinds of diabetes mellitus include: Cystic Fibrosis-related diabetes, different kinds of Monogenic Diabetes, Congenital Diabetes, due to genetic defects of insulin production, and Steroid Diabetes, induced through high doses of glucocorticoids.

Type 1 Diabetes mellitus

This type of diabetes requires daily insulin injections or wearing an insulin pump to regulate levels.

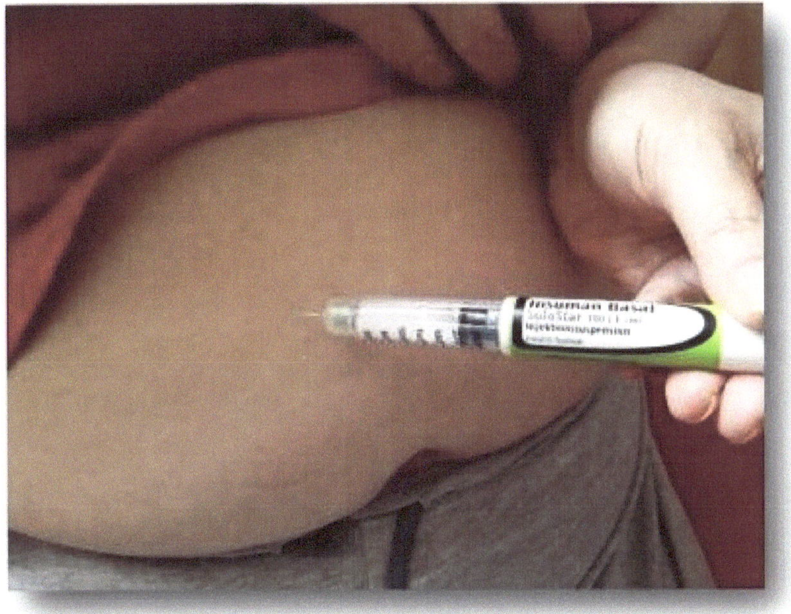

Type 2 Diabetes mellitus

Type 2 DM, results from an insulin resistance. In this condition, the cells fail to use the insulin produced by the pancreas correctly. This condition may also be combined with a complete insulin deficiency in some cases.

Gestational Diabetes

Gestational diabetes is a form that occurs in pregnant women. Often there is no previous diagnosis of diabetes and the high blood glucose level may return to normal after delivery.

In some cases, this may precede development of Type 2 DM; however, many women only require medication and monitoring for the duration of their pregnancy.

Managing Diabetes

Discovering that you have diabetes can be overwhelming and challenging news for many people. Keep in mind that this condition affects individuals of all ages and races. Many people are born with the disease, and other people develop it later in life.

You are not alone in managing diabetes. Take a deep breath and decide to take control of your diabetes, instead of allowing it to take control of you.

Incorporating exercise into your day, changing your eating habits and learning how to monitor your glucose levels will enable you to live a healthy and productive life. You can also make sure you get adequate sleep and reducing any stress will also help to keep your blood sugar in check. These can be monumental lifestyle changes for some individuals.

Be patient with yourself. Do not try to overhaul everything on the first day. Knowledge is power. The more calm and open-minded you can stay while you educate yourself about this new condition, the better off you and your loved ones will be.

Risk Factors for Diabetes and How To Be Proactive

Understanding the risk factors of diabetes will help you understand what kind of preventative measures you can take in reducing the associated risks that accompany this condition. Many people learn how to listen to their bodies with this disease. Often it provides the wake-up call a person needs about some much-needed lifestyle changes.

Other people, however, may go into denial about their condition. They may even rebel and decide not to take their medicine on time, or not to make time to check their blood sugar levels. These individuals often suffer dire consequences as a result. Instead of managing their disease, they allow it to progress and may end up dealing with numerous other health problems. Choose to be proactive and as healthy as you can. It is never too late to start making positive choices.

Obesity

Obesity is the largest risk factor for Type 2 diabetes. Unfortunately, obesity is at pandemic levels in many countries. This abundance of excess weight causes a lot of stress on the entire body. The joints, the cardiovascular system and the internal organs are all affected.

Many studies have been done to determine why obese people have a higher tendency to develop diabetes. One theory shows that abnormal glucose output is increased in obese people and the pancreas has a difficult time responding with the required amount of insulin.

It is possible to deal with obesity in a healthy manner. Start with small changes in your daily routine. Park your car at the farthest point from work or the store and increase your daily steps. Take the stairs whenever possible. Keep raw veggies in a bowl of water in the fridge for a nutritious go-to snack. Drink a glass of water before every meal to help convince your body that you feel fuller faster. Visit with a dietician who specializes in diabetes and learn some new recipes!

Sedentary Lifestyle

A sedentary or low activity lifestyle is another common diabetic risk factor. Keeping active and staying on your feet increases your blood flow and promotes healthy circulation. If you sit at your desk all day, make time to stretch and get some fresh air during lunch and coffee breaks. Are in the habit of watching TV after supper? How about choosing to go for an evening walk around the block instead? These small changes will have a positive impact on your overall health.

Diabetic Apps and Online Resources

Remembering to check your glucose levels and monitoring your blood sugar can be challenging for many diabetics. Thankfully, there are a variety of smartphone and tablet apps or applications in both android and iOS that you can download to help educate you on your journey with diabetes.

Some of these apps offer reminder alarms for taking medication or for checking blood glucose levels. There are other apps available that will monitor your exercise and your carbohydrate intake and offer built in medical terminology explanations. Other applications have suggestions for exercise, meals and tracking net carbs along with overall calorie intake.

Many of these apps offer comprehensive tools for either Type 1 or Type 2 diabetics.

For example, users of practically any age can organize all their data such as:

- medications

- insulin
- test
- diet
- glucose

... etc. required to improve and manage their condition. Many people utilize the ability to generate reports and graphs that can be shared via email with their healthcare professionals or printed out and logged at home.

Online Resources

There are a variety of free online tools available to help diabetics manage their health. Logbooks that can help keep track of medication intake, exercise regimes, blood pressure and glucose levels are often useful to help users track inputs and outputs and identify trends in their daily routine.

Community support combined with collaborative sharing to improve health and motivate positive changes are additional beneficial online tools.

Many glucometers come with a USB hook-up or have one available for purchase that will enable you to download information directly onto your computer. Speak with your doctor and local pharmacist to see what type of meter they recommend. Do some research and ask around.

Check in with your health insurance provider as many will cover your glucometer or test strips or at least a portion of your supplies.

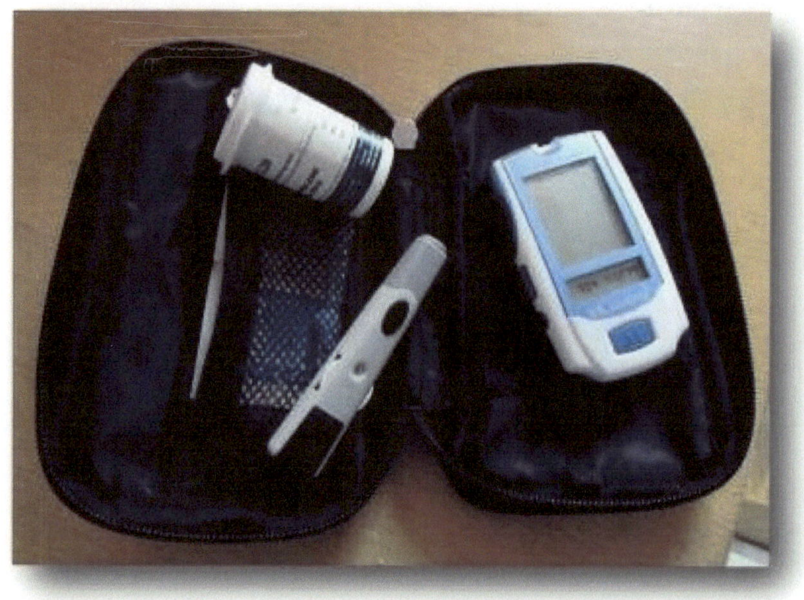

Online Support Groups

Feeling angry, guilty or in denial about having diabetes is commonly experienced by many individuals after they are diagnosed. You may find support from diabetes groups online. If you are having difficulty dealing with the stress, speak with your doctor as they may be able to help you.

As well as online support groups, there are often local support groups that can be a great place to connect with others who are dealing with similar issues. Your doctor can refer you to a dietician and a counsellor if needed too.

Insulin and Blood Glucose

Every person's blood contains sugar that is also referred to as glucose. Blood sugar is essential for human health. We obtain glucose from the foods we eat. The blood takes the role of carrying it into the different organs of the body to provide energy to the cells thus allowing the muscles to move, the brain to think and other important functions of the entire body.

Blood glucose is the fuel for normal body and brain function. But like most things in life, too much of a good thing can be a bad thing! Uncontrolled levels of blood sugar can have devastating and long-lasting, even permanent, effects on organs and tissue.

Maintaining Normal Levels of Blood Glucose

When talking about blood glucose, balance is the key. Although blood glucose is very important for the many processes that are taking place inside the body, its levels should not be too high or too low. Otherwise, the person becomes at risk of some serious health problems.

Fortunately there are many things that you can do in order to keep healthy levels of glucose in the body. Aside from regularly monitoring your glucose levels, which is a must if you have diabetes or at high risk of developing such condition, you also need to get a better understanding of how glucose behaves and functions to keep it functioning at an optimum level.

The Importance of Having Normal Levels of Blood Glucose

The human body has the innate ability to keep the levels of glucose high enough for the millions of cells to stay well nourished. The human body also has this natural scheme of preventing glucose from going too high to avoid it from getting in the way of many important biological processes that are necessary for keeping the body healthy.

To regulate the levels of glucose, the body needs the help of some other parts of the body including: the muscles, fat tissue, brain, liver, small intestines, pancreas and a variety of hormones including insulin.

However, when one or any of these glucose-regulating body parts do not function well for some reason, the individual may suffer from elevated levels of blood glucose, resulting in diabetes.

If left untreated, having elevated levels of glucose may damage the person's eyes, nerves, blood vessels, and kidneys, along with peripheral limbs like the feet.

How Blood Glucose Behaves Inside the Human Body

For people who do not have diabetes, their bodies can keep the levels of blood glucose within 70- 100 mg/dl. After eating, foods will be broken down for their nutrients to be used by the different parts of the body.

As the process of digesting the food is taking place, their blood glucose will temporarily increase. While the levels of blood glucose are increasing, the release of insulin is additionally being triggered by the pancreas to ensure that blood glucose levels do not get too high.

Insulin is a peptide hormone produced within the pancreas. It is released into the bloodstream to help regulate fat and carbohydrate metabolism.

Now, signals are being sent to the numerous cells inside the person's body, especially those that are found in their fat, liver and their muscles. Once the signals are received, these body parts will absorb the extra glucose to convert it into energy or store it in the liver as glycogen for future use.

Most of us have heard about insulin. In the past, we mostly hear about it in relation to those people affected with Type 1 diabetes. This condition requires those affected to inject insulin to survive. They also need to constantly monitor their sugar intake to better manage their condition.

Today, incidence of Type 2 diabetes far outstrips that of Type 1. Type 2 diabetes is rapidly becoming the greatest single disease risk in developed countries. The tragedy is that as it is a lifestyle disease, it is preventable.

What Is Insulin?

Insulin is a peptide hormone that is produced by the pancreas. Insulin signals the tissues in our muscles, fats and liver to extract excess glucose from the blood so it can be used for energy requirements or stored as glycogen, and ultimately bodyfat.

In a healthy person, eating a balanced diet, insulin is released on demand, in metered amounts to match the levels of glucose that the blood contains.

When the amount of glucose in the blood is within normal levels, the process of releasing insulin will either slow down or stop.

The foods that we eat and the beverages we drink each day directly impact insulin release in the body and can have profound effects on how we feel, how we perform, and on our short and long-term health.

Why Do We Need Glucose?

Our cells require glucose for their energy source. Our bodies cannot create our own glucose, so we rely on our food intake to obtain it. Much of what we eat has some glucose extracted from it during digestion.

Regardless of where it comes from, glucose obtained from our diets will end up traveling into the bloodstream so it can reach those tissues that need it.

The different chemical composition of different food types determines how much glucose is extracted from it, and how quickly that occurs as we digest the food.

Too Much is NOT a Good Thing

Simplistically it may seem that as we need glucose, the more the better, and the faster extracted the better. Unfortunately, the opposite is true, for two main coexistent reasons.

Firstly, our bodies evolved processing complex carbs, protein and fats.

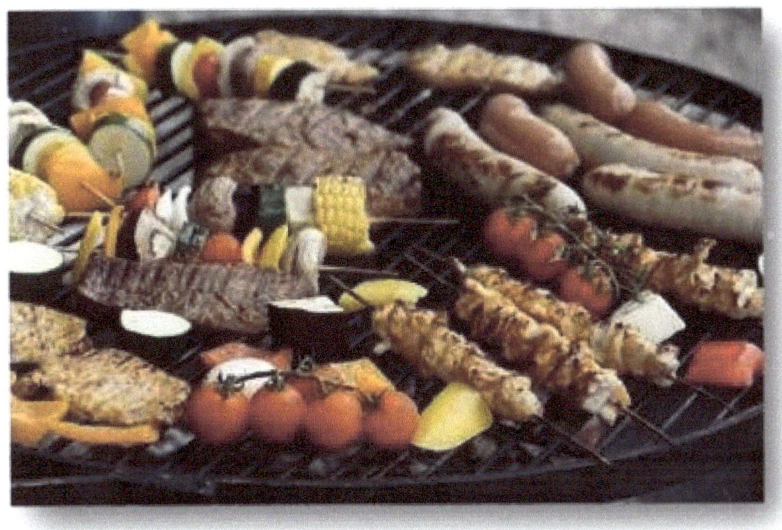

For our paleolithic ancestors, simple carbs were almost non-existent, certainly very irregular. Glucose release was steady, and all was used by energy demands. Diet problems related to lack of food.

Secondly, the reverse is true today. Diet problems revolve around too much rather than too little. Even more importantly, predominant food types have changed.

Far too much of many diets contain an excess of simple carbs, which flood our blood stream with glucose in amounts far more than our immediate energy requirements.

Not only is this excess dangerous, much of it is very quickly converted into bodyfat.

Carbs, Protein and Fats as Glucose Sources

Carbohydrates are most easily converted into glucose. Simple carbs are chemically little different from sugar, and easily and rapidly converted to glucose. Our saliva also contains enzymes that break down these simple carbohydrates even before they reach the stomach.

Complex carbs require more digestion than simple carbs to convert the glucose.

Proteins are converted into sugars through the process called *gluconeogenesis*. Fats are also being converted into glycerol derivatives and glucose.

Protein and fats yield much less glucose per gram of food than do carbohydrates, and also requires more digestive effort to break it down to release the glucose molecules.

High GI carbs contain higher volumes of simple sugars. These are broken down to blood glucose rapidly and can cause problematic or dangerous 'sugar spikes'.

Complex, low GI carbs and fats and proteins break down more slowly and are more safely handled by the body's metabolic processes.

This means that the glucose obtained from protein, fats and complex carbs are released at uniform, useable rates. In response, insulin only needs to be released at low levels to perform its vital tasks.

Insulin Panic Response

Conversely, when we consume simple carbs, from sweets, soft drinks, many processed foods, or anything else that contains sugar, our blood is almost immediately flooded with glucose.

As the body cannot utilize the flood of glucose immediately, this causes a panic insulin release, an insulin "dump", to sweep the excess glucose from the blood.

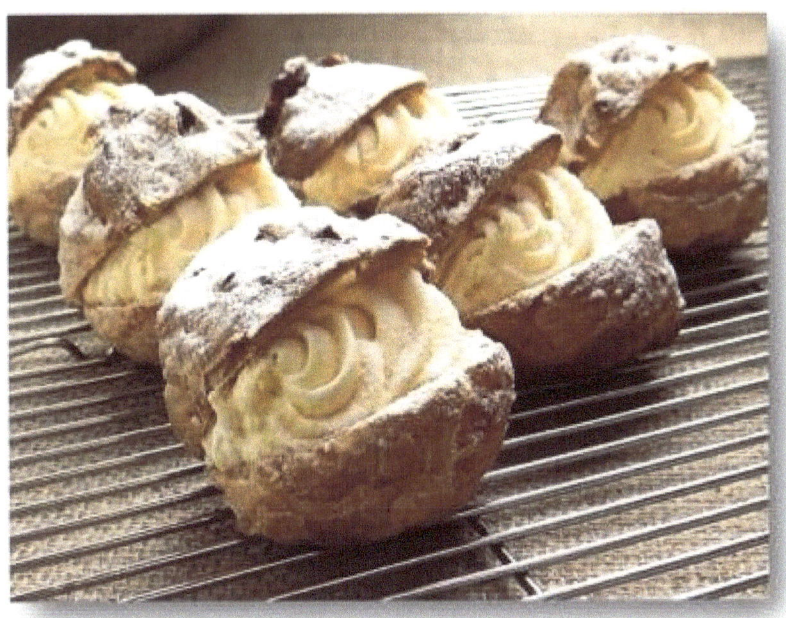

This is a critical body reaction as the high level of glucose in the blood is dangerous to many parts of the body. The insulin triggers cells to uptake the glucose, either to be used as an energy source or to be sent to the liver to be converted to fat for longer-term storage.

Type 2 Diabetes – Why Does It Develop?

If this occurrence is rare, the body can deal with it, however if high GI simple sugars are a constant component of a person's diet ongoing problems occur. Firstly, the body's cells become insulin-resistant, and require ever-increasing amounts of insulin to trigger a response.

In turn, the pancreas will tend to overcompensate by releasing larger amounts of insulin to cope with the excess glucose in the body, due to the failure of resistant cells to respond effectively, so insulin is released in ever-increasing amounts, more and more each time.

At a certain point, the body cells are so desensitized to insulin that the blood glucose stays in the blood for much longer than it should.

This is an extremely dangerous condition, and this is Type 2 diabetes!

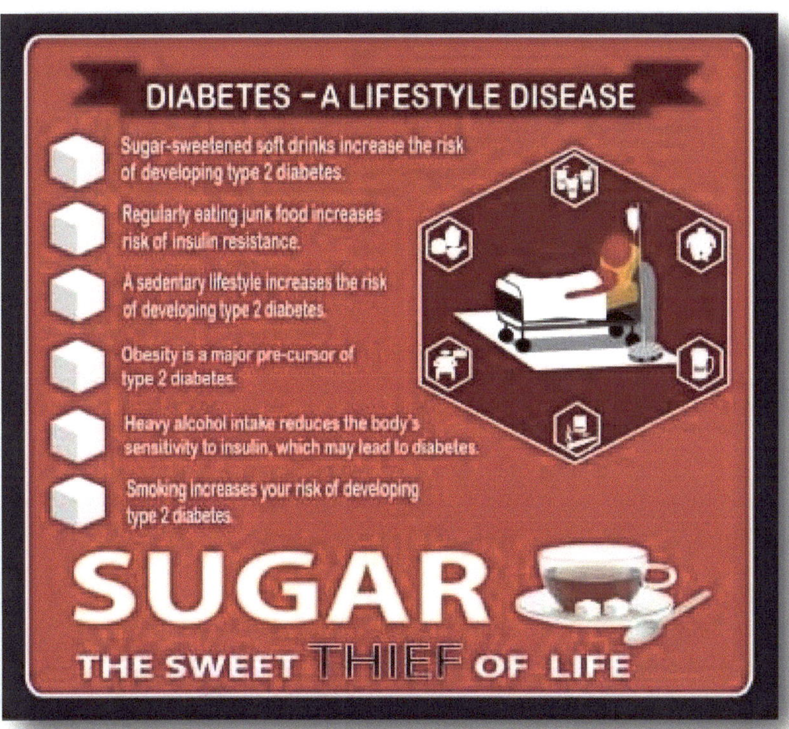

DIABETES – A LIFESTYLE DISEASE
Sugar-sweetened soft drinks increase the risk of developing type 2 diabetes.
Regularly eating junk food increases risk of insulin resistance.
A sedentary lifestyle increases the risk of developing type 2 diabetes.
Obesity is a major pre-cursor of type 2 diabetes.
Heavy alcohol intake reduces the body's sensitivity to insulin, which may lead to diabetes.
Smoking increases your risk of developing type 2 diabetes.
SUGAR
THE SWEET THIEF OF LIFE

Carbohydrate Cravings – a Big Diabetes Risk Factor

Pre-diabetes is a condition in which an individual's blood glucose levels are higher than the acceptable range but not high enough to be diagnosed as diabetes. Being given a diagnosis of pre-diabetes means essential changes to lifestyle (predominantly diet, but also exercise) *must* be undertaken immediately to prevent further progress towards Type 2 diabetes.

Weight gain and sedentary lifestyle greatly increases a pre-diabetic person's risk of developing Type 2 diabetes. Reducing weight now is no longer a matter of vanity, it is a crucial health concern.

A basic understanding of how Type 2 diabetes develops should give a realization that the problematic food type is carbohydrates, specifically simple carbs. One of the best ways to avoid gaining weight, and to reduce bodyfat, is teaching yourself to overcome your carb cravings.

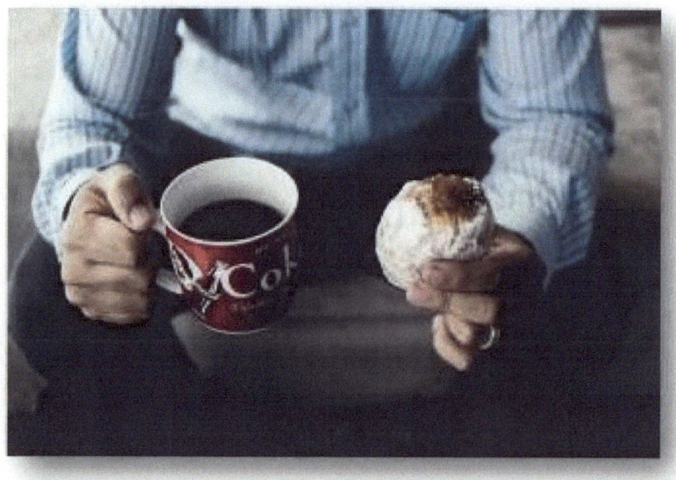

Things You Should Know about Carb Cravings

Many people's food cravings include French fries, chocolates, potato chips, soft drinks, pastries and cakes. Unfortunately, these foods are loaded with sugar, fats and sodium.

There is no doubt that these foods do taste so good they make an individual crave for more. Food manufacturers and processors are very aware of this, and use these ingredients to enhance their products. They are included because they taste good, not for their nutritional value.

A big part of avoiding Type 2 diabetes comes down to making adult choices – am I mindfully eating for my health's sake, or simply at the mercy of my taste buds?

Like every indulgence, cravings can become addictions and may eventually turn into a temptation that a person can hardly resist. Continuing to indulge in these tempting foods can be causing and adding to problems with your health.

Fats and Type 2 Diabetes

For preventing and overcoming Type 2 diabetes, fats are a preferable food source to simple carbs. In a healthy diet containing few simple carbs, fats are an excellent fuel source. However, if simple carbs are the dietary mainstay, some fats can exacerbate the problem. Avoiding the food types above will reduce consumption of both bad fats and simple carbs.

How to Resist Your Carb Cravings

Overcoming your carb cravings may seem to be a very challenging task but it is certainly possible. We have all received different advice in the past for breaking bad habits, but there some proven steps for dealing with changing food behaviors.

Planning, Not Willpower

Don't rely on willpower, that is setting yourself up for failure. Make realistic goals, action steps and plans and follow them always.

Determine your problem points when they occur. Instead of wallowing in guilt afterwards, analyze the situation and look backwards to the events preceding the point of failure. Make changes for next time so the issue does not re-occur, so that your willpower is not tested.

For example, the first thing that you should do is to make your house, car and office devoid of any temptations.

Stop putting cookie packages in the cupboard and cakes or sodas in the refrigerator. Seeing these foods in your kitchen or anywhere in the house will only turn on your brain's pleasure system which has become fixated on craving for these foods.

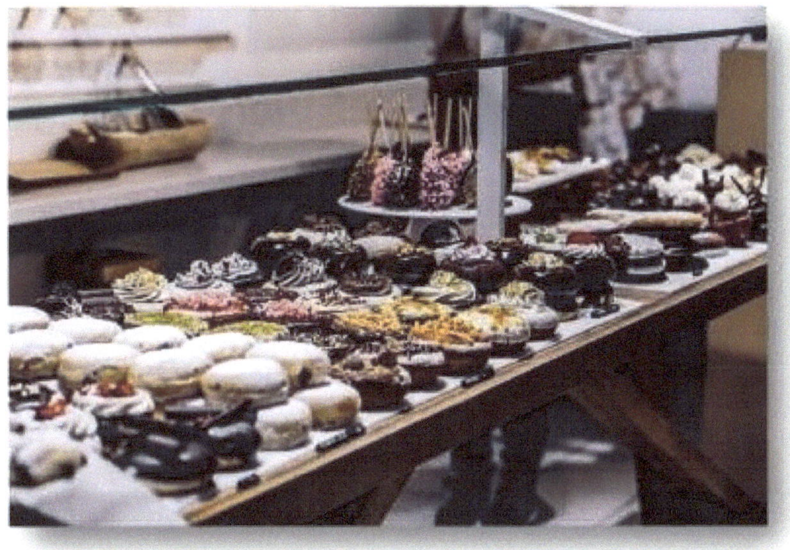

Change what you buy at the store, so you don't have them tempting you. Don't kid yourself that you will buy things you shouldn't 'just in case' or in case someone turns up for coffee or a chat. If they are there in front of you, they will be eaten at some stage.

Replace these food items with fruits, carrots, and nuts that are nutritious snacks to easily grab should your cravings haunt you again.

Don't shop for groceries when you are hungry!

Change Your Food Types

Our child-mind, the one that responds to taste temptations, has convinced us over time that only responding to our cravings can satisfy our hunger. This can lead us to limit our intake of better food types such as protein and healthy fats.

When you stop eating simple carbs and eat some protein at every meal, in a very short time you will be surprised at how you don't feel hungry all the time. This is a natural condition, it is how it meant to feel, but this feeling is taken away by a diet that is constantly based on sugary simple carbs.

Ditching these bad habits may entail a lot of failures in the beginning but with persistence you will find it easier to resist your cravings. After a while you will find the cravings are not there, unless triggered by exposure to the foods themselves.

Once you do decide on conquering your food cravings, be determined enough to follow it through. Care enough about yourself to make conscious healthy food choices for yourself, instead of letting your taste buds do it for you.

Studies reveal that those who are pre-diabetic can still prevent Type 2 diabetes by making a conscious effort to lose weight and eat properly.

Diabetic Diet – Healthy Meal Tips

Ideally, a diabetic diet consists of a high intake of lean meats, lots of vegetables and whole grains. Additionally, it is low in sugar, low in salt and low in simple carbohydrates. Just because you have diabetes does not mean that you must sacrifice your love of all richly-flavored and delicious foods. Many of your favorite recipes can be adapted to become a healthier version that your entire family will enjoy.

Healthy and Tasty Meal Tips

Don't know where to begin? Following are some tried and true suggestions for improving your diet.

These changes need not be sudden or dramatic, but adopting these practices so that they become the new normal for you and your family will provide a path to greatly improved dietary health.

Discarding Unnecessary Fat

Fatty cheeses and meats are known to increase the levels of cholesterol in the blood. This can greatly increase the risk of heart disease over time. Developing an increased risk of heart disease is one of the complications of diabetes and hyperglycemia.

A diabetic who regularly consumes fatty foods could greatly increase their risk of stroke or heart attack. A diabetic diet that focuses on protein sources which are low in saturated fats, such as beans, fish and lean meats is a much healthier option.

Grilling, broiling or barbecuing meats is an excellent way to reduce your fat content at mealtime. Utilizing non-stick cookware means you can still sauté your favorite dishes without adding extra fat.

Substituting some of the meat in your casseroles with brown rice, bulgur or tofu, will help you replace some of the meat in your diet with a lower fat option.

Another great trick is to allow your cooked stew, spaghetti sauce or soup to chill. This enables the fat to congeal on the top and you can easily scoop this layer off before reheating and eating. Baking in the oven with a rack over a drip tray is another simple way to remove fat while you are cooking and thereby keep your calories lower and your cardiovascular system healthier.

Steaming

Steaming vegetables and adding flavorful herbs to the water or broth during the steaming process can be a great way to enjoy your favorite colorful vegetables. To begin with; thyme, rosemary, sage and parsley are popular savory herbs that can spice up almost any meat, fish or veggie dish. Cinnamon, nutmeg and cloves are other herbs that you only need a pinch of to deliver a punch of flavor!

Vegetarian Night

Try making one night a week "vegetarian night". Meatless dishes can provide a great opportunity for you to be creative. Enjoy some marinated bean salads, experiment with quinoa or try a stir-fry with tofu. Vegetarian chili is another great option. Adding kidney beans and lentils to your favorite soups is another nutritious way to fill up. Indian style curry dishes may become a new family dish.

Discover New Cheese

Experiment with different cheeses. Using sharper flavors will allow you to use less in your dishes and enjoy stronger flavor. If you don't prefer the grease that often occurs from baking cheese, perhaps place some freshly grated on the table at meal time and people can sprinkle on for a tasty alternative.

Portion Control

To help you keep track of your portion size, work with the space on your plate. Substituting large supper plates with smaller dishes can dramatically reduce your portion size. Filling up a salad plate with supper for instance, will help you fill your plate with less food.

A well-balanced plate may consist of ½ vegetables, ¼ of proteins, such as fish or chicken and a ¼ starch, such as brown rice or quinoa.

If you top it all off with fresh fruit for dessert, you will have a satisfying and nourishing meal and won't feel like you are missing out on anything.

Exercise for Diabetics

If you are a diabetic thinking about starting a new exercise regime, it is a good idea to check with your doctor first. Getting into the habit of checking your blood sugar before, during and after your workout will also give you a clearer picture of how your body responds to increased physical activity.

Have a conversation with your doctor about how frequently you should be checking your blood sugars. Some people use their glucometer 6 times or more a day. Everyone is different. Speak with your doctor to see what they recommend in your particular case and follow their advice.

Understanding the way your body metabolizes glucose will help prepare you to pack the appropriate post-workout snack, especially if you are travelling to a gym or exercising outside of the home.

Incorporating exercise into your day is also a great way to relieve stress, not to mention of course, helping keep your body fit. Maintaining an active lifestyle will help keep your body functioning at its peak performance.

Physical Activity

Exercise lowers blood sugar levels. Studies have shown that exercise is comparable to medication which lowers blood glucose but with less side effects. People with diabetes still excel in sports and compete in competitions.

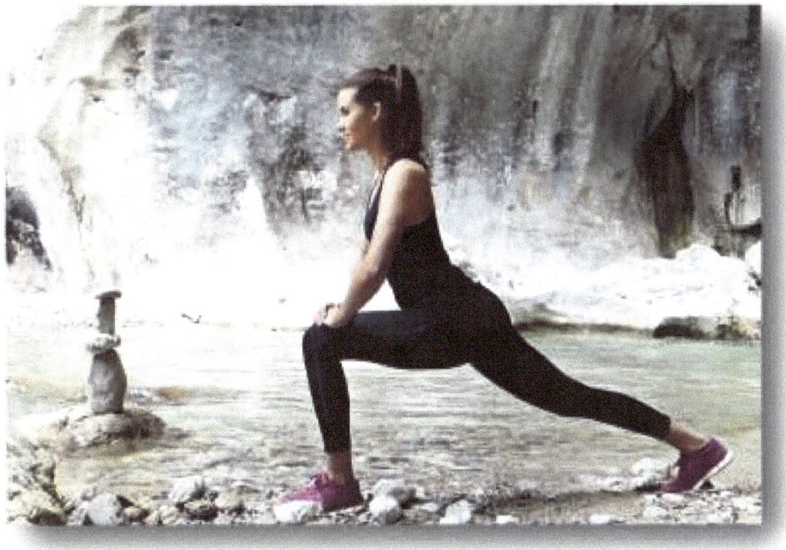

Having an active lifestyle and incorporating daily exercise is very beneficial to those living with this condition. Going for a bike ride, walk or swim each day can bring you a variety of health benefits. You do not have to sign up for an expensive gym membership to live a more active lifestyle.

Diabetes and Stress

Stress hormones are naturally produced in our bodies when we are under emotional or physical stress. Every person on the planet succumbs to these feelings on occasion. For diabetics however, stress can have an even greater negative impact on your total health.

Since stress can significantly raise the blood sugar levels in your body, it is important to find healthy ways to alleviate these emotions to avoid their consequences. Exercise is an invaluable option during these times.

Doing a quick set of push-ups, squats or shadow-boxing will help you release that pent up negative energy and burn up some potentially dangerous blood sugar. Often stressful situations can make us want to overeat or drink too much alcohol, both of which will increase blood sugar levels. Choosing to go for a brisk walk will be a much more beneficial coping mechanism. Low-impact exercises that protect your knees and your feet are also great choices.

Sensory Neuropathy and Foot Ulcers

Sensory Neuropathy is one of the main concerns that diabetics may have cause to deal with; particularly when it comes to implementing a new exercise routine. In this condition, the patient loses feeling in their feet due to the high glucose levels interfering with the electrical impulses in the nerves.

Symptoms including burning, coldness and tingling sensations, along with extreme sensitivity to touch are common. The loss of sensation and numbness can leave patients unaware that they have injured their feet.

Diabetics may severely burn themselves while stepping into a bathtub filled with hot water too! This is why washing the feet with ONLY warm water is strongly recommended. If the feet are not properly dried or if exercising in new shoes, chafing or blisters may occur. The open wound or sore on the foot may become infected if it is not healed quickly. Preventing infection is a top priority in this situation.

Disinfecting the wound with diluted tea tree oil will help keep it germ free and assist healing, plus wearing pressure relieving pads in the shoes can also be beneficial.

Exercising can do wonders to improve the health of those living with diabetes. Physical activities help the body respond more effectively to insulin and reduce levels of blood glucose.

Often, though not always, lack of exercise has contributed to succumbing to Type 2 diabetes, however diet is usually the major factor. Exercise works best when used in conjunction with a diabetic meal plan, especially in controlling Type 2 diabetes.

There are some diabetic cases, especially if advanced, that limit the ability to exercise. For many diabetics, mobility has become reduced, and the thought of exercise is not a palatable one.

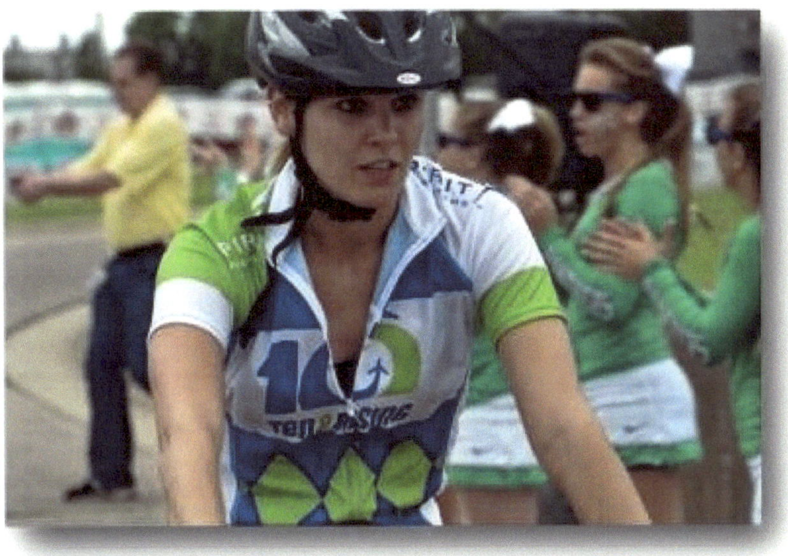

Exercise does not have to be strenuous, and for those who are profoundly unfit, it should not be. For most diabetics, light exertion will greatly aid their recovery.

Through exercising, an individual will be able to improve circulation especially in their legs and arms, which are common problem areas for people with diabetes.

Studies have shown that older people tend to have lower levels of insulin sensitivity. One reason for this is the reduced physical activity in the senior years. Staying active, or resuming after inactivity, will benefit an individual for life.

Safety Tips for Exercising

If you have been diagnosed with retinopathy, it is best to avoid exercise routines that require heavy weight lifting. Otherwise, you will be at risk of damaging the fragile blood vessels in the eyes. If you suffer from peripheral neuropathy, always choose durable but soft footwear.

If you have a history of heart attack or high cholesterol and triglyceride levels, it is highly recommended that you undergo a cardiovascular examination before deciding to start on any exercise program.

If your urine has ketones, or if you are experiencing pain, tingling or any discomfort in your legs, your doctor may recommend taking it extremely easy.

Recommended Physical Activities

Any aerobic activity that is done in moderate intensity may prove to be very beneficial for diabetics. These are the kinds of activities that allow the heart rate to increase and make the person sweat, without causing undue strain. If the exercise affects your ability to talk normally, back off the intensity a bit.

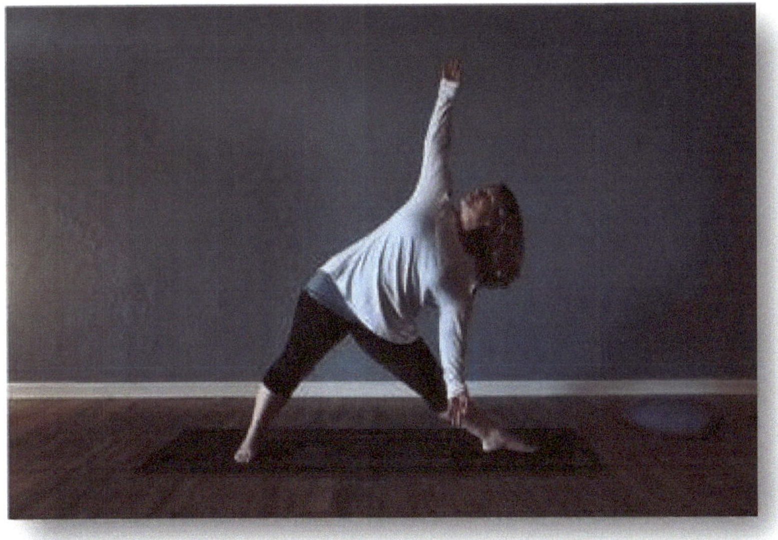

Popular physical activities include: fast-paced walking, bike riding, yoga, water aerobics and light jogging.

Exercise for Weight Loss

If you are exercising to reduce weight, it is important to remember that the body will call on ready-to-use blood glucose first. It will only start to metabolize and utilize fat reserves when excess blood sugar levels have been depleted.

If you eat or drink sugar-rich foods prior to or during exercise your body will release insulin, which in turn triggers the body cells to uptake or store the excess blood glucose. This is opposite to what you are trying to achieve.

Often this 'panic release' of insulin combined with exercise can result in a debilitating 'sugar slump', which can lead to feeling exhausted beyond what the exercise should have caused.

For more effective weight loss, avoid foods containing excess sugar.

How to Avoid Leg Cramps

Before going to bed, do a little exercise first, by stretching your calf muscles up to three times. Make sure that your legs are not tucked in too tightly under your sheets to avoid any constriction or difficulty in moving your legs while sleeping.

You may also increase the intensity and duration of your exercise regimen but you need to do it in a gradual manner.

Flexing your toes towards your knees may also help avoid leg cramps. However, if you find this too painful to perform, try grabbing your toes by flexing them slowly toward your knees.

It is also helpful if you gently massage your calf. Applying ice packs or hot compresses will also help your muscles to relax. Try both ice and heat therapy and see what feels best for you.

Here is the best cramp-prevention tip of all. Don't eat any simple carbs or starches after mid-afternoon. The very same foods that worsen your risk of Type 2 diabetes are a major cause of night cramps. If they persist, cut out starches such as bread, pasta, rice and potato as well.

Type 2 Diabetes and the Family

It can be stressful on the entire family when a diabetic diagnosis is confirmed. There are many things that need to be taken into consideration including learning how to cope with new dietary changes while being supportive and patient with the newly diagnosed family member.

This can be an especially worrying time, particularly if it is a child or a teenager who has been diagnosed. Children may be afraid of the lancets used for monitoring blood sugar levels. This is a huge lifestyle change for everyone and time to adjust is needed.

Reward kids for checking their glucose levels, but don't reward with food treats as this may add to the problem.

Involve the family in grocery shopping together and hunting for new diabetic-friendly recipes. Get everyone active and go for walks, swims or bike rides together.

Be patient with outbursts of denial or anger. Don't allow guilt to make your feel like "things may have been different if only..."

Learn how to take control of diabetes in a safe, educated and healthy manner and don't let it take control of you.

Diabetes Prevention - Helpful Eating Tips

Studies have shown that individuals, who have a high-risk of developing diabetes, significantly lowered their risk and prevented or delayed developing the disease after losing weight. The very best way to maintain a healthy weight is to enjoy a healthy diet. A healthy diet combined with regular exercise may be the best prevention against diabetes.

If your doctor finds you a high-risk candidate for diabetes, they may recommend you follow a specific meal plan that is tailored to your current nutritional needs. It is important that you eat three meals in a day and have appropriate snacks in between to maintain an optimal blood sugar balance. Skipping a meal is a big no-no for people who have diabetes or who are at risk. Keeping regular meal times will help you have better control over your blood sugar levels.

When eating, it is vital to be very aware of your portion sizes. You may need to research a bit about the right portion sizes for each food category. You may wish to ask your doctor or your dietitian about portion sizes and food servings to ensure that you are eating the correct amounts of the right foods.

Limit your intake of foods that contain high levels of unhealthy fats. You also need to be careful about cooking methods. For example, when you need to use oil, make sure to select the kind of oil that does not contain trans-fats or saturated fats.

Other foods that you should limit if not eliminate in your daily diet includes fatty portions of meat, whole milk and other dairy products that contain whole milk, fried foods, candies, crackers, cakes, pies, salad dressings, lard, and nondairy creamers. It is always better to opt for foods that are raw, boiled, broiled, grilled and steamed as they do not contain unhealthy fats.

Whole grain foods are a rich source of fiber. This can be found in cereals that contain 100% whole grains, oatmeal, and other foods which are made from whole grains such as bagels, pita, rice and tortillas. Other rich sources of fiber also include dried herbs, flax and sesame seeds, edamame, sun-dried tomatoes, beans and passion fruit.

Reduce Your Sugar Intake

If you are fond of reaching for a can of soda, then now is the time to start ditching that habit. It is a good idea to start getting used to drinking coffee without sugar in it and avoid those fruit-flavored drinks as well.

You may also want to ask your doctor or dietitian about healthy sugar substitutes. If you want to get rid of your craving for soda, try making your own fresh fruit juice.

Fresh fruit juice already tastes sweet and it does not have to be added with sugar to taste delicious. Your juicer can become your new best friend.

Be Conscious with Your Carb-Cravings

As a person who is at high risk of developing diabetes, you need to be aware of your carbohydrate intake as well. Carbohydrates can have a great impact on your blood sugar levels and this is the reason why you need to be conscious about the amount of carbohydrates that you consume on a daily basis.

You may ask for help from a dietitian about measuring food portions. If you are not already doing so, aim towards becoming well-educated about reading food nutritional labels when you are shopping. Particularly pay more attention to portion sizes and the amount of carbohydrates that each food product has.

A healthy diet is ideally coupled with regular exercise. Ask your health care provider and your fitness expert before starting any exercise regimen.

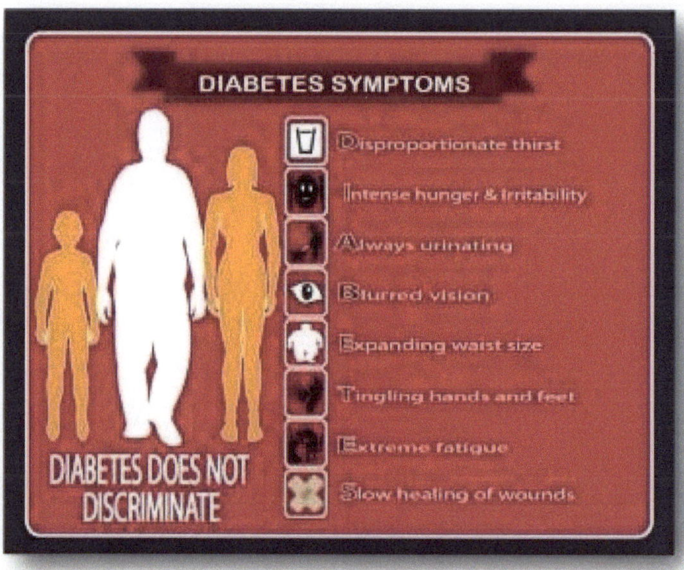

Complications and Herbal Supplements for Diabetes

There have been more than 400 different traditional plant medicines documented for treating diabetes. Few of these plants have been studied for their efficiency, although, in undeveloped countries they are often the main choice for non-insulin dependent diabetes.

Under no circumstances should children or adults who are insulin dependent discontinue their insulin injections. Herbal treatments may be used after consultation with your family doctor. If you do implement any dietary supplementation, it is wise to advise your doctor of any changes so they can have all the facts when monitoring your health.

Certain minerals such as: Zinc 25mg; Chromium 50mcg-125mcg; Magnesium 300mg; and Manganese 15mg have been useful to help glucose metabolism normalize. Note that mg stands for "milligrams" and mcg for "micrograms".

Other helpful supplements include: Vitamin B6 and B-Complex, Brewer's yeast and Vitamins A, C and D. Brewer's yeast naturally contains chromium and this mineral assists in the metabolism of sugar.

Some popular herbs for reducing sugar in the urine include: Sweet Sumach, Pipsissewa, Olive leaves, Jambul seeds and onions. Bitter Melon and Balsam pear have also been used successfully. Guar gum has been used in hyperglycemia to reduce the sugar in the blood.

Where the pancreas is still functioning, hypoglycemic herbs can be effective. Popular hypoglycaemic herbs used to raise blood sugar levels include: Goldenseal, Dandelion root, and German Chamomile.

Additional "anti-diabetic action" herbs include: Goat's Rue, Bilberry berries, Fringe Tree, Fenugreek seeds, Aloe Vera and garlic.

Diabetic Neuralgia

Cayenne pepper has been successfully used for Diabetic Neuralgia. There are creams containing the active ingredient capsicum that may be applied and capsules are available for internal consumption. Cayenne is beneficial for increasing the circulation and this can be beneficial for some of the cardiovascular side effects of diabetes as well.

Diabetic Gangrene

Tinctures with equal parts of Echinacea and Thuja have been very helpful for this necrotic condition. The tincture can be taken internally, 30-60 drops and also rubbed externally onto the affected area.

Blindness, Glaucoma and Detachment of the Retina

Developing cataracts is a common occurrence in diabetes. Although surgery may be necessary, herbs can be supportive for these issues. Preventative checkups with the eye doctor and related health care specialists are the best defense for this complication.

Heart Disease and Kidney Strain

Coronary Heart Disease is common in diabetics. Women in particular need to be proactive so as not to develop atherosclerosis at an early age. Taking essential fatty acids can greatly benefit the heart and the cardiovascular system. They can help lower triglyceride levels and bring high blood pressure down. High blood pressure unfortunately can place extra strain on the kidneys. The kidneys may become exhausted from excreting too much protein. Lime flowers, Hawthorn and Yarrow can be helpful for this situation.

Foot Ulcers

Feet that are exposed to unconscious bruising and chafing may develop an injury from which septic ulceration may occur. Chamomile foot baths are a very soothing and healing treatment that can be easily done at home. Remember to check the temperature of the water before soaking the feet.

Final Thoughts

These guide does not intend to offend anyone and is not judgmental in any way. If anything it contains caused you offense, ask yourself why. Don't let past repeated behaviors be a justification for maintaining your status quo, if that is a place you don't want to be, health-wise.

It is possible to prevent Type 2 diabetes and even overcome it, depending on the degree, however, changes will need to made to your lifestyle. The same eating behaviors that caused the problem are not going to fix it.

Be your own best friend and take the advice you would give to someone you really care about, and follow it to a diabetes-free life.

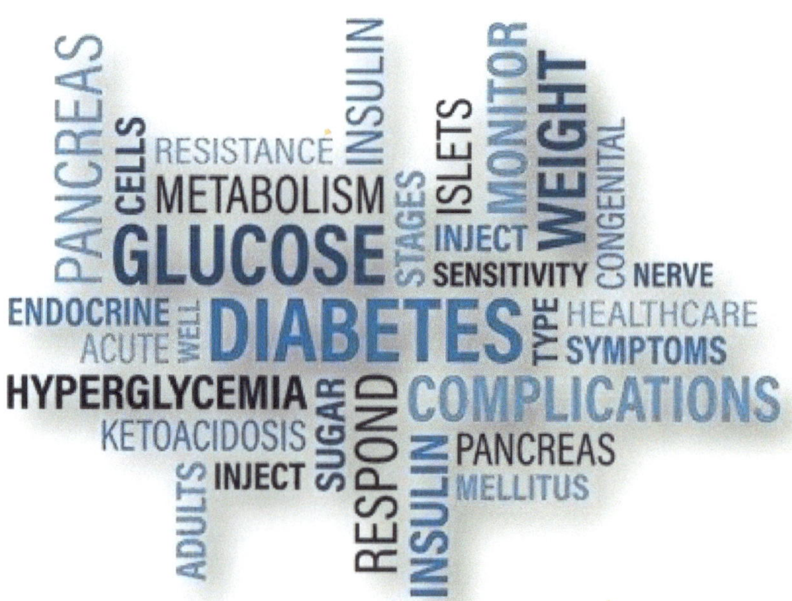

About the Author

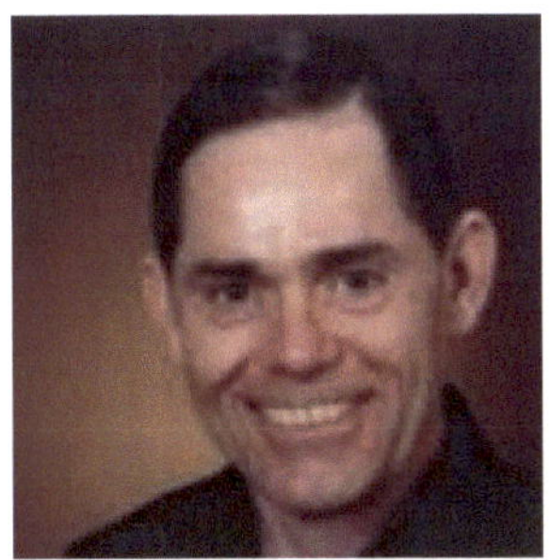

I have published over 125 books on Amazon for Kindle, CreateSpace and other publishing platforms.

While most of my books are on health and fitness in general, as I age (now 65) at the time of this writing) my topics of interest are geared toward aging baby boomers and older.

Besides my own writing, I also ghostwrite ebooks, books, reports, articles, blogs and do Kindle conversions for clients on a variety of topics.

Today my wife and I are retired from our careers and live in Gold Canyon, AZ. I now write as a retirement business where you'll find me happily sitting in my office typing away on my laptop as I work on my next book or ghostwriting project . . . that is if we are not traveling on a cruise ship - our new-found mode of travel.